Quit coffee

Short table of contents

It looks as if your body and cells have forgotten that there is coffee in the world.

No caffeine withdrawal symptoms... Will you become a "superman" due to a finer perception of your surroundings?

Dear reader,

I translated the original Hungarian text into your language using Google Translate. I tried to write in such a way that it would translate as error-free as possible. If somewhere the text is not well understood, I apologize.

- I haven't had coffee in months.
As a result, I feel much better, and the condition of my body has also improved.

-Before, I was quite a coffee drinker: the first thing I did in the morning after getting up was to sip a mug of coffee.

- It was very good.
Later, approximately
I had an espresso around 8 o'clock.
Then one to the south.

Then maybe another 1 at half past 3-4
in the afternoon, it was simply good.

-When drinking coffee in the
afternoon, I noticed several times the
feeling that I didn't really need the
coffee: The sugar content of the cake
with the coffee, that's what my body
needed.

- The obsession with having
afternoon coffee...

- At that time, I didn't even think that one day after a program I would suddenly stop drinking coffee from one moment to the next.

 - I couldn't even imagine how this could be possible...

 (In 2023 I read an article in a newspaper that predicted that in about 50 years there will be less and less coffee-growing regions on earth due to global warming.

- Then I briefly thought about what it would be like without coffee, but I came to the conclusion that it will no longer affect me).

-Since I stopped drinking coffee regularly, I haven't felt any disadvantages.

-Neither mentally nor intellectually.

- Since then, much more positive things have happened to me...

(My wallet was better).

- What happened is that my body, like a bio-machine, simply exists, exists, works, constantly at a very good level, there are no major constraints, "to have a coffee first...".

- In addition, I can perceive the currents, waves and other people coming towards me from the outside world much better than before.

- Often subtle things that those around me don't yet perceive, but I already know.

-Strangely, the body can perceive many things better in its normal state without the internal acceleration.

-Years ago, I noticed a strange thing happening in my body suddenly when I drank coffee:

- Many times after drinking an espresso without cream and sugar, I felt that the coffee was like a roasted seed when it entered my stomach, - my body sent me the stimulus many times that "I have received poison, they want to poison me".

- That's why my body, my body's sensors suddenly got scared.

 Through this fright, they came to the present, so to speak, and suddenly began to perceive their surroundings better, lest the body die.

 -The body avoids danger.
-This is the moment when one's perception will improve after drinking coffee.
This has happened to me several times.
- Now I will introduce you to the program.

- Will you be shocked when you see how this is related to quitting coffee?!

The program lasts for 3 days apple juice cure.

For 3 days, you only drink freshly squeezed apple juice.

You don't eat anything.
You don't drink coffee in the morning.

 - You only drink apple juice.

You'll make it, I've done this program several times, I made it too.

-The original purpose of this program is to cleanse your body and liver.

- This works so well in this program that the various substances deposited in the cells will be washed out of your body and cells.

Of course, coffee grounds too,
- because of which a person is forced to drink coffee again and again.

The cells are, so to speak, "drugged", and if some "toxin" remains in the cell, the cells will start asking for that drug again after a while.

- In this case, the coffee, and you feel that "I should drink a coffee", - or because my blood pressure has dropped.

- When the body gets scared after drinking coffee,
-"what kind of poison did I just drink?"- as a result, your attention units start to work better, but that requires higher blood pressure...

 Therefore, the body quickly starts an "emergency program", which also increases the blood pressure.

 -In today's world, you can already be told to imagine your body with an artificial intelligence (which is a drug addict), but you are the boss of your body.

This program lasts for 3 days.

The day you start the program, you stop drinking coffee from that morning.

 You only drink delicious apple juice for 3 days.

It's really delicious.

Get a fruit juicer and about 15 kilograms of delicious apples.

 It can be sweeter, but there should also be some sourness in it.

 - I always did this program on weekends, Friday-Saturday-Sunday.

- On Monday, it's good if you're near the toilet, because the apple juice can still cause you to have sudden diarrhea.

- Don't buy apple juice in the store, it's not freshly squeezed, it also contains additives, - don't fool yourself.

Don't copy working technology.
Buy real apples, about 15 kilograms.

You will be a little hungry, but bearable.

 -Think about how much people were starving a few hundred years ago and endured.

You can last 3 days too.

 -During these 3 days, do not go anywhere and be near a toilet, because you will have sudden diarrhea from about the 2nd day.

(Even the bowels will be well cleaned from the inside by the diarrhea).

 You will see for the result that it is worth it.

So you take the fruit centrifuge, centrifuge the juice of one or two apples and sip it slowly.

Depending on the size of the apple, the juice of 1 or 2 apples will be enough for 1 glass.

(You don't do it in advance with several glasses, the reason is that, for example, bite into an apple, then put it down, and after about half an hour look at the bite mark: it will turn brown.

 - Oxidized in air.

The apple juice needs to oxidize in your stomach and intestines.
It's better for your body).

Here are the times when you drink apple juice:

At 8 o'clock: 1 glass.
(2.-2.5 deciliters).
at 10 o'clock: with 1 glass.
At 12 o'clock: with 2 glasses.
at 2 p.m.: with 2 glasses.
4:00 p.m.: 2 glasses.
at 6 p.m.: with 2 glasses.
at 8 pm: with 1 glass.

Sip it. for 3 days.

In the meantime, you don't eat anything.
You only drink apple juice. You can handle it.
Apple juice has enough energy and water content that your body needs.

- My observation is that the body cleansing effect of this treatment really begins to work on the 3rd day.

 - On the morning of the 4th day, you can have a good breakfast.

One of the phenomena of the apple juice cure: the body will be so clean that it does not need coffee afterwards.

- I have already observed several times after the apple juice cure that on the morning of the 4th day, when the 3-day cure was already finished, my body did not ask for coffee on the morning of the 4th day.

 - It is interesting that I, as a being in the body, asked for coffee. Just out of habit.

- This came from my time trace, from previous lives.

 -But this stimulus can be changed with a decision, you just have to decide that I, as a being, don't need coffee either.

-This attitude works. I haven't had coffee in months.

Result:

Since I stopped drinking coffee, after the apple juice diet, several positive things have happened in my life:

On the morning of the 4th or 5th day, when I looked in the mirror after getting up, I suddenly realized that I had become more beautiful.

 -I, the 63-year-old old man, said this to myself when I saw myself in the mirror: "Well, I'm prettier!".

- This is so true that I even wrote a book about it.

- My senses are refined.

-I can imagine this refinement of the senses as the cells asking for the coffee before the apple cider. The cells begin to emit a kind of subtle vibrations of desire, waves of desire. You notice that they are asking for coffee because it is your stimulus, your inner desire that you should drink a coffee.

-On the other hand, you also perceive your environment as if you are "taking the broadcast".

So you perceive the other vibrations flowing towards you from your environment, - that's how you receive the broadcast.

But for this your cells should be in a resting state.

-If your cells tremble for coffee or other things, then they cannot perceive a lot of waves and vibrations coming towards you from outside due to their tremors and vibrations.

This will make your perception duller.

After the apple juice meal, the body does not need coffee.

The coffee residue was washed out of the cells.

The cells, within the cells, do not have a molecular amount of coffee residue, which would cause them to ask for more coffee.

The cells behave as if they have forgotten that there is coffee in the world.

I didn't experience any coffee withdrawal or caffeine withdrawal symptoms.

Since your cells no longer emit "desire waves" after the apple juice cure, your body and cells can also sense the finer waves coming into the body from the outside.

-Try it, you'll notice it after a while.

You yourself will notice that a little
You have become a "super human".

Wild animals also have good
perception because they do not
consume drugs, so their bodies and
cells are better able to perceive their
environment, the vibrations and
waves flowing towards them.

(It is also possible that your
environment will say about you after
a while: "How the hell does He know
all this?").

-In addition, your whole body will be
cleaner from the inside.

You will feel much better, you will be more mobile.

In addition, you will notice a lot of positive changes in yourself.

This could be presented well as if you have a car that you have been using for years, the car has several faults, but you know them and you can handle the car with these faults, you are used to it.

 But suddenly you get into a new car and it has no faults, so you suddenly feel the difference between the new car and the old car.

In the morning, for example, drink
tea, or eat an apple instead of coffee,
or muesli. Be resourceful.

(It is possible that even alcohol can be
weaned in this way, - I don't drink, I
don't know - but I do know that after
the 3-day course, the body does not
need foreign substances. I would do
this program with an alcoholic over
several weekends in a row , until his
body is completely cleansed.
 Then I would decide with him,
that He, as a soul in his body, what is
the point of his alcoholism.
-Don't drink alcohol, only the
perception of reality is disconnected
from alcohol, and you still have
friends even if you don't drink.

He doesn't have to drink because
those around him also drink and
expect him to drink too).

-Dear reader, I will finish my thought
process, I hope you will be able to
quit coffee with this program, if that
is why you bought this brochure.

I have been doing this apple juice
cure regularly for about 8 years, 2-3-4
times a year, as I feel like it.

I don't remember if I could have
stopped drinking coffee even after the
first time, - that was not my goal at
the time.

If you're doing it because you want to stop drinking coffee, but it doesn't work after the first course, then repeat the course, then it will definitely work.

Do this treatment 2 or 3 times a year, as you like.

- Maybe even your smile will be more beautiful, because your teeth won't turn yellow from coffee.

As an afterword, I have to say that coffee is also an article of pleasure.

If a man takes away from himself all kinds of articles of pleasure, then why does he live?

-However, your perception will be better.

Well, you know, but the above description works, I wrote my own experience.

Please, if you bought this booklet as an E-book, buy it also in paper form, the reason is that the E-book may disappear after a while, but the paper form will remain on the shelf and you can show it to others later.

Good luck,
Best regards:

Keszthelyi Sándor

© 2024 Sandor Keszthelyi
Herstellung und Verlag:
BoD – Books on Demand,
Norderstedt
ISBN: 9783759768124

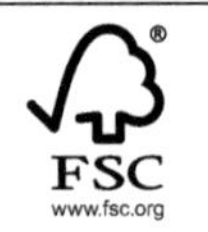
FSC
www.fsc.org
MIX
Papier aus ver-
antwortungsvollen
Quellen
Paper from
responsible sources
FSC® C105338